Public Health in the 21st Century

Types and Causes of Childhood Diarrhea

PUBLIC HEALTH IN THE 21ST CENTURY

Additional books in this series can be found on Nova's website under the Series tab

Additional E-books in this series can be found on Nova's website under the E-books tab.

PUBLIC HEALTH IN THE 21ST CENTURY

TYPES AND CAUSES OF CHILDHOOD DIARRHEA

TINUADE A. OGUNLESI

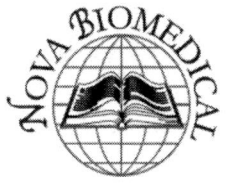

Nova Science Publishers, Inc.
New York

Copyright © 2010 by Nova Science Publishers, Inc.

All rights reserved. No part of this book may be reproduced, stored in a retrieval system or transmitted in any form or by any means: electronic, electrostatic, magnetic, tape, mechanical photocopying, recording or otherwise without the written permission of the Publisher.

For permission to use material from this book please contact us:
Telephone 631-231-7269; Fax 631-231-8175
Web Site: http://www.novapublishers.com

NOTICE TO THE READER

The Publisher has taken reasonable care in the preparation of this book, but makes no expressed or implied warranty of any kind and assumes no responsibility for any errors or omissions. No liability is assumed for incidental or consequential damages in connection with or arising out of information contained in this book. The Publisher shall not be liable for any special, consequential, or exemplary damages resulting, in whole or in part, from the readers' use of, or reliance upon, this material.

Independent verification should be sought for any data, advice or recommendations contained in this book. In addition, no responsibility is assumed by the publisher for any injury and/or damage to persons or property arising from any methods, products, instructions, ideas or otherwise contained in this publication.

This publication is designed to provide accurate and authoritative information with regard to the subject matter covered herein. It is sold with the clear understanding that the Publisher is not engaged in rendering legal or any other professional services. If legal or any other expert assistance is required, the services of a competent person should be sought. FROM A DECLARATION OF PARTICIPANTS JOINTLY ADOPTED BY A COMMITTEE OF THE AMERICAN BAR ASSOCIATION AND A COMMITTEE OF PUBLISHERS.

Library of Congress Cataloging-in-Publication Data

Available upon Request
ISBN: 978-1-61728-168-6

Published by Nova Science Publishers, Inc. ✛ New York

PUBLIC HEALTH IN THE 21ST CENTURY

TYPES AND CAUSES OF CHILDHOOD DIARRHEA

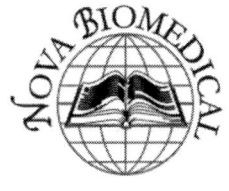

Contents

Preface		vii
Introduction		1
Chapter I	Diarrhoeal Syndromes	3
Chapter II	Epidemiology of Diarrhoea	5
Chapter III	Mechanisms of Diarrhoea	7
Chapter IV	Predisposing Factors	9
Chapter V	Aetiology of Watery Diarrhoea	11
Chapter VI	Dysentery	19
Chapter VII	Persistent Diarrhoea	27
Chapter IX	Chronic Diarrhoea	29
Conclusion		33
References		35
Index		49

Preface

The three clinical types of childhood diarrhoea include - acute watery, persistent and dysentery. Acute watery diarrhoea which lasts for less than 14 days constitutes 60 to 80% of childhood diarrhoea while persistent diarrhoea lasting for more than 14 days forms 3 to 12% of all cases. The presence of blood in diarrheic stool makes it dysenteric and this occurs in 10 to 20 % of cases in the developing world.

Childhood diarrhoea may be secretory, osmotic or invasive. Most cases of childhood diarrhoea in the developing world are infective. Close to 90% of enteropathogens in childhood diarrhoea are identifiable particularly with serology. Enteropathogens may be viruses, bacteria or parasites. These pathogens may exist singly or in combination. Rotavirus accounts for 25% to 65% of severe diarrhoeal diseases requiring hospitalization. Other viruses include Norwalk virus, Norwalk-like virus and the enteric adenoviruses. Bacterial agents may account for close to half of all cases of childhood diarrhoea in the community in the developing world. Enterotoxigenic *Escherichia coli* (ETEC) is the most frequently isolated bacterial cause of acute watery diarrhoea. Others include *Shigella, Campylobacter, Yersinia, Salmonella* and *Vibrio cholerae*. Parasites commonly associated with watery diarrhoea include *Entamoeba histolytica, Giardia lamblia, Ascaris lumbricoides, Enterobius vermicularis* and *Trichuris trichuira*. It is important to note that only the presence of vegetative forms of *E. histolytica* and *G. lamblia* confirm the pathogenicity of these organisms.

Most cases of persistent diarrhoea are associated with *Escherichia coli, Campylobacter, Shigella, Giardia, Aeromonas* and *Cryptosporidium*. *Shigella dysenteriae* had been reported to account for more than 60% of dysenteric cases, *Campylobacter* for 5% and *Entamoeba histolytica* for less than 3% of cases. There are recent evidence that *Entamoeba histolytica* may be more frequently associated with childhood dysentery in the developing world than ever known.

Chronic diarrhoea is uncommon and mostly encountered in situations of severe immunosuppression or metabolic and endocrine disorders. In HIV/AIDS, the etiology of chronic diarrhoea include enteropathy caused by direct viral invasion of the gut epithelium or infections caused by *Cryptosporidium*, *Microsporidia*, *Isospora belli* and Mycobacterium Avium Complex. Less common in the developing world are malabsorption syndromes associated with tuberculous enteritis, zinc deficiency, pancreatic insufficiency, lactose intolerance, milk protein intolerance, abetalipoproteinaemia and Celiac disease. Hyperthyroidism, the carcinoid syndrome and scleroderma are associated with abnormalities of gut motility resulting in diarrhoea.

In conclusion, the etiologies of childhood diarrhoea appear to vary in different locations on the globe.

Introduction

Diarrhoea is a leading cause of childhood morbidity and mortality globally. It is estimated that under-five children may experience up to 1.3 billion diarrhoeal episodes per child-year and this may be associated with 4 million deaths particularly in the developing world. Available data suggest that diarrhoea is associated with childhood deaths globally. It forms 16.3%, 12.7%, 19.5%, 14.0%, 16.7% and 12.0% of all under-five deaths in the African, American, South East Asian, European, Eastern Mediterranean and Western Pacific regions of the world respectively as at 2004 [1].

The World Health Organization defines diarrhoea as the passage of 3 or more loose or liquid stools per day, or more frequently than is normal for the individual [2]. Faecal consistency is determined by the quantity of water it contains. A single explosive watery stool or unusually frequent but formed stools may be abnormal and must not be ignored although such do not conform with the standard definition of diarrhoea. For breastfed newborn and young infants, frequent passage of loose stools may be completely normal due to the effect of the gastro-colic reflex, yet it is to pay attention to what the mother of an infant considers abnormal.

Chapter I

Diarrhoeal Syndromes

There are three major clinical diarrhoeal syndromes in childhood: acute watery diarrhoea which starts abruptly, the frequently passed stool does not contain visible blood and lasts for less than 14 days [3]. Indeed, most cases of acute watery diarrhoea subside within 7 days. It must be distinguished from dysentery which also begins acutely and the diarrhoeic stools contain visible blood. Persistent diarrhoea begins acutely and lasts longer than 14 days. It may start either as watery diarrhoea or dysentery [3]. While acute watery diarrhoea is the commonest type of childhood diarrhoea, persistent diarrhoea is the least common [1,5,6]. Dysentery forms between 7.7% and 30% of all childhood diarrhoea cases in different parts of the developing world [6-9].

Chronic diarrhoea is a term loosely used to describe long-lasting diarrhoea. The definitions adopted for this disease entity varies in different studies. It has been variously described as diarrhoea lasting for more than two weeks [2], four weeks [10] and six weeks [11]. Nevertheless, adopting fourteen days or two weeks in defining chronic diarrhoea may be confusing with respect to persistent diarrhoea with which it is also interchangeably used. However, the major difference lies in the fact that chronic diarrhoea is often of non-infectious origin [2].

Chapter II

Epidemiology of Diarrhoea

The incidence of diarrhoeal diseases is highest in children under twenty four months [12] and especially between six and eleven months [13]. The reasons proposed for this pattern include poor immune status and poor weaning practices especially with poorly nutritive, bulky and heavily contaminated foods [15].

It is estimated that more than three quarter of diarrhoeal deaths occur in children less than two years of age [16]. This is because of the higher fluid turn-over rate which puts them at a higher risk of developing severe fluid and electrolyte deficit during diarrhoeal episodes.

In Mexican children with dysentery, *Shigella* was found to be more common (35 %) in those between 1 and 5 years than among infants (10 %) [17]. The isolation rates of *Salmonella* and *Campylobacter* have also been reported to be higher in infancy than at any other time in childhood [17]. Parasitic diarrhoea appears uncommon among infants while the prevalence increases with age [18,19]. On the other hand, the prevalence of rotavirus diarrhoea decreases with age being highest in infancy [20,21].

Seasonal variation in diarrhoea incidence exists due to differences in climatic conditions. Isolation of *Shigella* was commoner in the dry season as reported from India [22]. This may be attributed to scarcity of water and the tendency to consume water from contaminated sources at that time of the year. The isolation of *Campylobacter* and *Yersinia* were also higher during the rainy season in Egypt [23] and Nigeria respectively [24]. Seasonal variations in the incidence of parasitic diarrhoea is however, not distinct since intestinal parasitic infestations are endemic in the tropics and subtropics [25].

Chapter III

Mechanisms of Diarrhoea

Intestinal physiology, with respect to fluid and electrolytes balance, includes two major processes: secretion and absorption. Of the over 120ml/kg of fluid that is secreted in to the gut on a daily basis, 95% is reabsorbed over the entire surface of the small and large intestine such that the net intestinal fluid loss in stools is less than 5ml/kg/day. This is strictly balanced on the secretory and absorptive functions mediated by the cellular transport systems in the epithelial lining of the gut. The Sodium-Potassium Adenosine Triphosphatase (ATPase) pumps sodium out of the cells into the blood vessels thus, creating a concentration gradient between the lumen and the epithelial cells. Sodium moves from the gut lumen into the enterocytes along with water. The sodium-coupled glucose transport, sodium-coupled amino acid transport and the sodium-hydrogen exchange pump are other active transport mechanisms involved in the process of absorption. On the other hand, intestinal fluid secretion occurs by active transport of chloride ions into the gut lumen [26].

Homeostasis is maintained by balancing intestinal fluid secretion with absorption. The balance may be disrupted by decrease in absorptive surface area from extensive villous damage, abnormal intestinal motility and chemical-mediated excessive fluid secretion. Therefore, diarrhoea results when there is net fluid loss into the lumen such that stool production is greater than 10g/kg/day. For clinical purposes, diarrhoea is described in terms of increased stool fluidity and increased frequency of passage. Increased stool fluidity makes it loose or watery. Loose stools are described as stools which take the shape of the container.

The pathological types of diarrhoea are described as follows: [27]

(i) Secretory diarrhoea. Certain substances within the intestinal lumen facilitate increased chloride secretion by the intestinal crypt cells. Exotoxins produced by organisms like *Vibrio* species and the Enterotoxigenic *Escherichia coli* (ETEC) stimulate the adenyl cyclise enzyme which increases the intracellular concentration of cyclic Adenosine Monophosphate (cAMP). This agent stimulates chloride secretion along with sodium and water and also inhibits chloride absorption. The resultant effect is increased luminal fluid followed by diarrhoea. The stools are voluminous and diarrhoea persists during fasting.

(ii) Exudative disease. Pathogens possess special characteristics for invading the intestinal epithelial lining thereby causing ulcers of various grades in the epithelium. The resultant effect is purulent bloody diarrhoea and the stools characteristically contain numerous pus cells. This diarrhoea persists during fasting and the stool volume is variable.

(iii) Malabsorption. Poor absorption of substrates may result from lack of digestive enzymes or lack of villous absorptive surface area. This leads to voluminous, bulky and pale stools of high osmolality. The diarrhoea persists during fasting.

(iv) Osmotic diarrhoea. This results from the presence of intrinsically non-absorbable solutes in the intestinal lumen. The effect of this is the creation of an osmotic gradient between the lumen and the epithelial cells. Thus, there is net movement of water out of the epithelial cells into the lumen causing luminal distension and diarrhoea. The stools are scanty and acidic. The diarrhoea stops during fasting.

(v) Increased motility with decreased intestinal transit time. This may be caused by the activity of specific hormones, chemicals and drugs which increase intestinal peristalsis.

Chapter IV

Predisposing Factors

Diarrhoea is prevalent or the epidemics tend to occur in places where sanitation and sewage disposal practices are poor, water supplies are inadequate or polluted and child feeding practices allow food contamination [28,29]. This is because most of the pathogens associated with diarrhoea are transmitted faeco-orally through contaminated foods, water and soiled fingers. An inverse relationship between the incidence of childhood diarrhoea and family's socio-economic status had been reported in a cohort of Nigerian children [30]. Poverty, ignorance and poor sanitation are characteristic of the lower socio-economic status hence, the higher likelihood of enteric infections. The specific factors predisposing children to diarrhoeal diseases include the under-listed:

1. Inadequate breastfeeding – breastfeeding protects children against enteric infections through the activity of secretory Immunoglobulin A, other immunoglobulins and antibodies, macrophages, lyzozymes etc contained in breast milk. Poorly breast-fed infants have been shown to be at higher risk of diarrhoea [31].
2. Poor waste disposal – House flies breed where refuse disposal is poor [32]. These insects act as vectors for most enteropathogens transporting them from improperly disposed sewage to food and water.
3. Poor personal hygiene (especially poor hand washing) – Enteropathogens are transmitted when materials contaminated with faecal matter are handled. Hand washing will be poor in the absence of adequate supply of clean water and the prevalence of diarrhoea is usually high in such places [33].

4. Malnutrition – Poor immune response is characteristic of malnutrition and this allows colonization and infection of the gastrointestinal tract by pathogens. Repeated gut infection leads to diarrhoea. Other salient features of malnutrition which predispose to enteric infections include decreased production of secretory Immunoglobulin A, decreased gastric acidity, altered gut flora and lactose intolerance following villous atrophy [34].
5. Exposure to fomites like feeding bottles – Bottle feeding in under-resourced parts of the world increases the risk of gastrointestinal infections due to extreme difficulty in adequately cleaning the utensils. Bottle feeding also reduces breastfeeding and impairs the protection potentially offered by breast milk and breastfeeding against pathogens.

Chapter V

Aetiology of Watery Diarrhoea

Most cases of childhood diarrhoea in the developing world are infectious. The infectious causes of childhood diarrhoea are mainly viral and bacterial and there is a recent emerging significance of parasitic causes of childhood diarrhoea.

Efforts have been repeatedly made to determine the role of identifiable pathogens in the causation of childhood diarrhoea. Interestingly, the results of such studies varied widely at different places and at different times within the same location. In places where access to medications is unrestricted, indiscriminate antibiotic use among children with diarrhoea may also influence the isolation of bacterial pathogens in diarrhoeic stools [35,36]. The isolation rate may vary from 40% to 84.5% or higher as shown in Table I.

The differential role of viruses, bacterial and parasites also vary. Table II shows the isolation rates of classes of enteropathogens in different parts of the developing world.

Hitherto, viruses were regarded as the most common causes of childhood diarrhoea in the developed world while bacteria predominate in the developing world but lately, viruses are also reported to be common in the developing world. This may be related to the availability of appropriate diagnostic facilities in the developing world. As shown in Table II, there appears to be a reversal of the role played by viruses with the most recent report from Ghana. Overall, 8% to 73.3% of diarrhoea may be viral [6,7,19,39,42], bacterial pathogens may account for between 4.8% and 52.2% of childhood diarrhoea [6,42,44] while parasites may be responsible for between 4.9% and 82% of childhood diarrhoea [6,18,42].

Apart from varying epidemiological factors, the likelihood of identifying pathogens in diarrhoeal stools is also hinged on the efficiency of the laboratory methods employed. Since the introduction of serological methods like the immunofluorescent assays, the enzyme linked immunosorbent assays or the polymerase chain reaction in the laboratory investigation of diarrhoea, the isolation rates of enteropathogens in diarrhoea has increased remarkably in most parts of the developing world where diarrhoea occurs commonly. Yet, no study has reported 100% isolation rate for enteropathogens in diarrhoeic stools. This may suggest other non-infectious aetiological factors in childhood diarrhoea. Diarrhoea may also occur as part of systemic illnesses like measles, pneumonia, septicaemia and malaria. This implies that it is imperative to conduct a detailed clinical evaluation for every child that presents with diarrhoea rather than restrict clinical attention to localized enteric infections.

Table 1. Overall isolation rates of enteropathogens in childhood diarrhoea in different countries

Location	Year of report	Isolation rate (%)
Ethiopia [37]	1982	70.0
Korea [38]	1989	75.8
Nigeria [39]	1994	74.9
Brazil [40]	2001	40.7
Colombia [41]	2006	84.5
Ghana [42]	2007	76.5
Burkina Faso [43]	2009	41.2

Table 2. Prevalence rates of viral, bacterial and parasitic aetiologies of in different countries

Location	Year of report	Bacteria (%)	Viruses (%)	Parasites (%)
India, China, Myanmar				
Mexico and Pakistan [7]	1991	48.0	23.0	3.3
Nigeria [39]	1994	59.1	26.5	2.3
Bangladesh [6]	2003	39.0	8.0	82.0
Ghana [42]	2007	4.8	73.3	4.9

Common Infectious Causes of Watery Childhood Diarrhoea

Rotavirus

This virus is a major cause of diarrhoea particularly among infants and young children. It is also the leading cause of diarrhoea requiring hospitalization among children. The prevalence rates of rotavirus among children with diarrhoea varied between 22.3% and 59.1% in Nigeria [18,21]. Local variations in prevalence rates of rotavirus are known and this may be related to the laboratory method applied. Prevalence rates as low as 5.2% had been reported in Bangladesh [6] as well as rates as high as 54.7% in Ghana [42]. The isolation rate was reported to have increased from about 21% over the 1981 to 1984 period to about 56% over the 1998 to 2000 period in Vietnam [45]. This apparent increase in rotavirus admission has been related to significant decrease in parasitic and bacterial diarrhoea admissions as a result of improved sanitation. The transmission of bacterial and parasitic agents is directly related to environmental sanitation unlike rotavirus which is transmitted either by direct contact or through droplets.

Rotavirus has been reported to co-exist with other viruses like enteric adenovirus [20,46,47] and other bacterial and parasitic pathogens [12]. The prevalence of rotavirus diarrhoea is highest in the first 24 months of life especially in late infancy [7,20]. The clinical significance of rotavirus infection lies in its tendency to cause fever, vomiting and severe dehydration requiring hospitalization [47]. Therefore, most diarrhoeal deaths in childhood are caused by the rotavirus [45].

Other Viruses

Less common viral causes of childhood diarrhoea include the enteric adenovirus, astrovirus, picorna virus, Norwalk virus and Norwalk-like virus. These agents may also co-exist with rotavirus [47]. Adenovirus commonly replicates in the epithelial lining of the respiratory and gastrointestinal tracts but only the serotypes 40 and 41 have been aetiologically associated with childhood watery diarrhoea. The prevalence of adenovirus serotypes 40 and 41 in childhood diarrhoea ranged from 3.8% to 9% [20,46]. Similarly, the prevalence of astrovirus in childhood diarrhoeic stools ranged from 1.2% to 7% [49,50].

Escherichia Coli

This is the leading bacterial cause of diarrhoea particularly in childhood [48]. The diarrhoegenic subgroups include the Enteropathogenic *E. coli* (EPEC), Enteroinvasive *E. coli* (EIEC), Enterotoxigenic *E. coli* (ETEC), Enterohaemorrhagic *E. coli* (EHEC) and Enteroadherent *E. coli* (EAEC). These organisms cause diarrhoea through different mechanisms hence, their contribution to childhood diarrhoea and clinical importance varies greatly. As a group, the isolation rate of *E. coli* in childhood diarrhoea ranged from 5% to 23% [41,51–53]. EPEC had been reported to be the most common bacterial cause of childhood diarrhoea in some studies with prevalence rates reaching 32.8% to 58.4% [44,54]. In some other studies, ETEC was severally reported to be the leading cause of bacterial diarrhoea among children in up to 20% of identified bacterial pathogens [38,39,48,55,56]. EIEC and EAEC are less common with prevalence rates ranging between 0.8% and 7% [52,56] and from 5.5% to 25% [40,52,57] respectively.

EPEC is widely known to cause outbreaks of watery diarrhoea in nurseries in the developed world but may cause persistent or chronic diarrhoea in the developing world [58]. ETEC is a common cause of secretory diarrhoea with the tendency to cause severe dehydration. Strains of ETEC produce exotoxins: the heat-labile toxins (LT) and/or the heat-stable toxins (ST). Studies have shown that most strains of ETEC produce ST (45% to 50%), LT (25% to 30%) and both LT and ST in 20% to 25% of cases [48,59]. These toxins cause excessive secretion into the intestinal lumen resulting in intestinal distension, hypermotility and severe diarrhoea. EIEC causes invasive diarrhoea very similar to shigellosis. It may cause severe dysentery and poses a major risk for persistent diarrhoea and malnutrition. EHEC produces Verotoxin which is similar to Shigatoxin produced by certain strains of *Shigella dysenteriae* type-1. This toxin is associated with extensive endothelial and epithelial damage resulting in haemolytic uraemic syndrome [60]. EAEC is associated with both acute and persistent diarrhoea in the developing world.

Shigella

This organism is known to cause infections that are mainly limited to the gastrointestinal tract. There are four clinically relevant species: *S. dysenterieae*, *S. flexneri*, *S. sonnei* and *S. boydii*. The most clinically important species is *S. dysenteriae* which causes severe watery diarrhoea and dysentery. This species produces an exotoxin which affects both the gastrointestinal tract and the central nervous system. This toxin, known as the Shiga toxin, produces voluminous non-bloody diarrhoea which later evolves into dysenteric illness following the invasion of the gut by the organism. The exotoxin can also cause meningism, seizures and coma [61]. The exotoxin is also known to cause haemolytic uraemic syndrome as a complication of shigellosis [60]. The other species are more likely to cause watery diarrhoea and persistent diarrhoea than dysentery.

The isolation rate of *Shigella* species in diarrhoeic stools ranged between 0.8% and 10.6% [41,51,62]. *S. flexneri* had been variously reported to be the leading *Shigella* species in watery diarrhoea with prevalence rate ranging from 3.8% in Bangladesh [6] to 6.1% in Brazil [40].

Salmonella

This organism causes enteric and systemic infections. *Salmonella enteriditis* and *S. typhimurium* are common causes of enterocolitis and but rarely cause bacteraemia. These organisms are associated with both watery diarrhoea and dysentery which may evolve into persistent diarrhoea. The prevalence rate in childhood diarrhoea varied between 2.1% and 24% [52,62–64].

Campylobacter

Campylobacter jejuni and *C. Coli* are the two common strains of this organism which are associated with both enteric and systemic infection. There is significant difficulty in distinguishing between the clinical disorders caused by the two strains. Similarly, ill-equipped laboratories may have difficulty differentiating between *C. jejuni* and *C. coli*. *Campylobacter* species typically cause acute watery diarrhoea, dysentery and persistent diarrhoea [65,66]. It was the most common enteropathogens in a cohort of Thai children with dysentery between 1998 and 2000 with a prevalence rate of 28% [67]. In that report, 80% of the Campylobacter species were *C. jejuni* while the remaining 20% were *C. coli*. In watery diarrhoea cases, reported identification rates for *C. jejuni* in watery diarrhoea ranged between 0.8% and 13% [37,41,42,63]. Indeed, some studies reported the absence of this organism in diarrhoeal cases [40,48].

Yersinia

These organisms are also known to cause all forms of diarrhoea in children. Both *Yersinia enterocolitica* and *Y. pseudotuberculosis* are known to cause diarrhoea either from the effect of enterotoxins produced by the organisms or from direct gut invasion. The isolation rate of *Yersinia* species ranged between 0.8% and 2.7% [39,40,43,68]. Some studies also reported complete absence of this organism in childhood diarrhoeic stools [37,42]. A remarkable variation in the species of *Yersinia* associated with childhood diarrhoea is known. In a cohort of Iraqi children, the isolation rate of *Yersinia* species was 1.6% and 75% of the isolates were *Y. enterocolitica* while 25% were *Y. pseudotuberculosis* [69]. Similarly, all the *Yersinia* species isolated in a cohort of Iranian children were atypical: *Y. intermedia* and *Y. frederiksenii* [68].

Aeromonas

These organisms produce enterotoxins which are postulated to cause diarrhoeal diseases. These are relatively common causes of childhood diarrhoea as the reported prevalence rates of the organisms in childhood diarrhoea varied from 0.5% to 9% [6,56,63,70]. In Nigeria, *Aeromonas hydrophilia* was reported among 0.7% to 3% of childhood diarrhoeal cases [39,71,72].

Plesiomonas

These organisms are relatively uncommon in childhood diarrhoea in the tropics. It was isolated among between 0.3% and 4% of children with diarrhoea [6,70,73]. None was reported in a Nigerian study [39].

Vibrio

Vibrio cholerae is known to cause severe episodes of watery diarrhoea which may occur in epidemics. The isolation rates of *Vibrio* species in sporadic cases of childhood diarrhoea varied from 0% to 0.5% [6,37,42,55,70]. The main subgroups responsible with the epidemics are the El-Tor O1 and O139 serogroups. Other species like *V. parahemolyticus* also cause less severe enteric infections. *V. cholerae* produces a heat labile enterotoxin which is responsible for prolonged hypersecretion of water and electrolytes into the gut lumen resulting in severe diarrhoea, severe dehydration, shock, renal insufficiency and death in a short period. Interestingly, *Vibrio* infections may also be asymptomatic as previously reported among children without diarrhoea [7,48,70].

Entamoeba Histolytica

A protozoan which exists either as the cyst, the intermediate precyst or the vegetative form (trophozoites). *Entamoeba dispar* is the lumen dwelling non-pathogenic commensal species of the organism while *E. histolytica* is the invasive species which causes enterocolitis, dysentery and hepatic disease. The isolation rate of *E. histolytica* in diarrhoeic stools of children ranged from 5.8% to 15.3% [6,18,53,57,64,74]. In Bangladesh, 3.8% of *E. histolytica* antigen-positive stools were watery while 0.92% was dysenteric. Similarly, only 7% of *E. histolytica* antigen-positive stools contained visible blood while 25% contained occult blood. This highlights the need to search for occult blood in stools in defining invasive enteric infections [75].

Giardia Lamblia

This flagellate inhabits the duodenum and jejunum. The cysts are excreted in stools of asymptomatic persons. However, the trophozoites may irritate the epithelial lining of the small intestine causing inflammation and acute or chronic diarrhoea. Children and immunocompromised adults commonly present with the features of giardiasis like abdominal pain, flatulence, bulky, greasy, foul-smelling stools in addition to watery or persistent diarrhoea. *Giardia lamblia* is a common parasitic cause of childhood diarrhoea with isolation rate ranging from 3.7% to 12.4% [18,41,42,76].

Cryptosporidium

These parasites are associated with mild, self-limiting diarrhoea in the general population but may cause severe chronic diarrhoea in immunocompromised individuals particularly with underlying HIV infection

[77,78]. The prevalence rate of this parasite in childhood diarrhoea ranged between 0.4% and 17.1% [6,18,42,64,76].

Common Non-infectious Causes of Childhood Watery Diarrhoea

Nutritional defects like acrodermatitis enteropathica (Zinc deficiency), pellagra (Niacin deficiency), Folate deficiency, fructosaemia and food allergies. These are characterized by various degrees of intestinal mucosal damage and inflammation.

Childhood poisonings may be associated with toxin-mediated hypersecretion and intestinal inflammatory changes. Such changes may occur following the ingestion of preformed exotoxins of *Staphylococcus aureus*, *Vibrio parahemolyticus* and *Clostridium perfringes*. Other poisons which may precipitate diarrhoea include iron and mushrooms.

Immunologic defects like combined immunodeficiency syndrome, hypogammaglobulinaemia, Immunoglobulin A deficiency and Wiskott Aldrich syndrome. These result in poor intestinal protection and recurrent enteric infections resulting in diarrhoea.

Endocrine defects like thyrotoxicosis, adrenogenital syndrome, Addison disease and hyperparathyroidism. These may be associated with increased gut motility and excessive intestinal fluid secretion.

Neoplastic conditions like neuroblastoma, pheochromocytoma and carcinoid syndrome may be associated with the secretion of vasoactive intestinal peptides. These substances increase intestinal secretions and motility [79].

Chapter VI

Dysentery

Compared with children who had acute watery diarrhoea, children with dysentery were relatively older, had higher frequency of stooling, lower frequency of vomiting, lower iincidence of dehydration and shorter duration of illness [80]. Dysentery is an invasive diarrhoeal disease with different degrees of intestinal mucosal damage ranging from ulceration to necrosis and loss of blood into the gastrointestinal lumen. Therefore, the presence of blood in diarrheic stools is taken as diagnostic of dysentery rather than the presence of mucus [81]. Dysentery is an important cause of morbidity and mortality that are associated with diarrhoea in childhood. In the developing world, it is estimated to cause about 10 to 15% of diarrhoeal episodes in under-fives and about 15% of all diarrhoeal deaths [1]. Specifically, dysentery formed 7.7% of all diarrhoeal cases in Bangladesh [82] but 24.2 % of diarrhoea in India [83].

Bloody diarrhoea may result from infectious and non-infectious, inflammatory diseases. The infectious form of this disease, also known as dysentery, occurs in two epidemiological forms: sporadic and epidemic. It may also be described as bacillary and the amoebic types depending on the aetiology.

Bacillary Dysentery

The commonest and most important causes of bacillary dysentery are the *Shigella* species. *Shigella dysenteriae* type-1 is known to cause most of the epidemic out-breaks of dysentery in Central and Southern Africa while *S. flexneri* causes the sporadic forms [84,85].

In terms of prevalence, *S. flexneri* appears to be the commonest specie in developing countries causing mild, self-limiting dysentery whereas *S. dysenteriae* type-1 which occurs in regional epidemics, causes the most severe forms of the disease [86].

Shigella causes about 60% of all dysenteric episodes, especially when the illnesses are clinically severe [87,88]. Apart from dysentery, *Shigella* may also cause watery diarrhoea as suggested by findings in the study done in Bangladesh in which 70% of confirmed *Shigella* infections presented with dysentery and about 30% as watery diarrhoea [7].

Salmonella species like *tyhimurium, choleracaesuis* and *enteritidis* are known to commonly cause acute enterocolitis and dysentery in man [89]. These species cause non-typhoidal salmonellosis as distinct from *S. typhi*, which causes the typhoidal form. The prevalence of Salmonella dysentery in most developing countries is generally low [90]. The prevalence varies between communities probably depending on the level of sanitation. Studies in Nigeria for example, have shown varying prevalence of salmonellosis. The prevalence of *Salmonella* may vary between 0.9% and 5.3% among under-five children with diarrhoea [25,91].

Campylobacter jejuni causes 5 to 15% of diarrhoea among infants worldwide [86]. In Harare [92], *Campylobacter* was found to cause 13.6% of diarrhoea respectively among children less than 24 months of age. In a study of a cohort of Thai children aged 1 to 12 years, Campylobacter was the leading bacterial cause (28%) along with *Shigella* (9%), *Salmonella* (18%), *Plesiomonas shigelloides* (1%) and EIEC (0.6%) [67]. Similarly, in a study of *Campylobacter* diarrhoea in Malaysia, 51% were dysenteric [66].

Yersinia enterocolitica infection is an uncommon cause of childhood dysentery [93]. It was found among 0.4% and 1.4% of cases in northern Jordan [94] and eastern Nigeria [24] respectively.

Enteroinvasive *Escherichia coli* (EIEC): This was isolated in 1% and 1.5% of childhood diarrhoeal cases in northern Jordan [94] and Calcutta, India [95] respectively. The other serotypes of *E. coli* are very rarely associated with dysentery.

Tuberculous enterocolitis may also manifest with passage of bloody stools or as culture negative chronic diarrhoea [96]. It causes ulcers on the mucosal lining of the terminal ileum which are characteristically transverse with undermined edges.

Clostridium difficile: Bloody diarrhoea caused by this organism usually follows recent or current antimicrobial therapy, especially when they are administered orally [97]. It is thought that antibiotics reduce the population of normal flora favouring the growth of *C. difficile*. The toxins produced by this organism produce the inflammatory changes in the intestinal mucosal lining, especially the colon [97].

Parasitic Dysentery

The commonest form of this is the amoebic dysentery caused by the *Entamoeba histolytica* [98]. Hitherto, this was believed to be rare among under-five children but common among older children and adolescents [86]. Some of the other species of amoebae usually found in the human gut but which are not pathogenic include *Entamoeba dispar, E. coli, E. gingivalis, E. hartmanni, E. polecki, and E. moshkovskii*.

About 10% of the world population is infected with *Entamoeba histolytica* and only 10% of these develop invasive disease like dysentery [99]. *E. dispar* is more prevalent than *E. histolytica* but it is only associated with the asymptomatic carrier state whereas the latter is the principal pathogenic species [99]. It was found among 4.9% and 5% of children with diarrhoea in northern Jordan, [94] and India [23]. The reported prevalence rates also depend on the method of diagnosis. For instance, higher rates were obtained in an Indian study with the use of serological methods, among children with and without diarrhoea [100]. This is important because serology may remain positive for quite some time after the acute illness has resolved and may, therefore, not be reliable in defining the current status.

The prevalence rates of *E. histolytica* were 50% and 35% among Nigerian children with diarrhoea and malnutrition respectively [101]. The 80.5% prevalence of *E. histolytica* among a cohort of Nigerian children was unusual [36] since previous reports of prevalence less than 3% are known [7,48].

Trichuris trichiura (whipworm) exists in warm climate and the excreted eggs may survive for 2 to 4 weeks in sewage. It formed 2.4% of childhood dysentery among Nigerian children [36] and 3.3% among children in northern Nigeria [102].

Non Infective Causes of Dysentery

The commonest non-infective cause of bloody diarrhoea in children is intussusception which is the in-folding of a portion of the gut into another segment caudal to it. About 60% of intussusception occurs among infants [103]. The exact aetiology is unkown but predisposing factors include viral infections with enlarged Peyer's patches, Meckel's diverticulum, parasitic infestations, intestinal polyps and haemangioma.

The other less common non-infective causes of bloody diarrhoea include the inflammatory bowel diseases like ulcerative colitis and Crohn's disease [104,105]. These are idiopathic chronic intestinal inflammatory disorders characterized by intermittent remissions and relapses. They are uncommon among Africans and Asians especially in infancy and are thought to have a strong genetic basis [106]. The initiating event is largely unknown but inflammatory mediators like cytokines, prostaglandins and free oxygen radicals are suspected to be involved. Ulcerative colitis is characterized by chronic inflammation of the epithelial layer with frequent passage of bloody, loose or watery stools associated with tenesmus and urgency.

Pathogenesis

The microbes causing invasive diarrhoea may either cause watery diarrhoea from toxin-mediated abnormal fluid secretion or from exudation which follows direct colonic epithelial invasion by the organisms.

Shigella

These inhabit only the human gut and are transmitted faeco-orally. The colonic invasion by *Shigella* is mediated by either the plasmid encoded traits or by chromosomally encoded factors [107]. Antibodies to the plasmid coded antigens have been demonstrated in human colostrum and breast milk and this may explain why *Shigella* infections are not common in children who are less than six months old and are on exclusive breastfeeding [108]. Shigatoxin, the exotoxin produced by *S. dysenteriae* type-1 and certain *E. coli* species known as the Shigatoxin producing *E. coli* (STEC) [109] as well as the Shiga enterotoxin-1 (ShET-1) produced by *S. flexneri* type-2a are specific chromosomal factors [109]. Shigatoxin stimulates intestinal mucosal

mast cells to release Leukotriene-C4, leading to the massive inflammatory response typical of *S. dysenteriae* infection.

The mechanism by which *Shigella* enters the epithelial cells of the gut may involve the invasion plasmid coded antigens (Ipa) [110] which binds to vinculin, a focal adhesion protein on epithelial cell surface. This increases the association of vinculin with F-actin and subsequent depolymerization of actin filaments and cytoskeletal rearrangements allowing phagocytosis at the site of bacterial entry. The phagocytotic vacuole is lysed and this is followed by infiltration by polymorphonuclear cells, disruption of membranes, cell death and tissue necrosis [111]. This mechanism results in ulcerations, microabscesses, exudation and increased stool liquidity.

Salmonella

The organisms can survive in sewage, dried foods and faeces for several weeks, hence, they are transmitted faeco-orally. Most non-typhoidal salmonellosis follows contact with contaminated animal products rather than from human contacts [89]. When it invades the ileal epithelium, it causes diffuse mucosal inflammation with erosion and microabscesses resulting in watery diarrhoea and dysentery depending on the degree of mucosal involvement.

Campylobacter

The spread of *Campylobacter* is usually by dogs and chicken and the organism invades the ileal and colonic epithelium by the actions of its cytotoxins and heat-labile enterotoxins. This organism has been reported to cause dysentery and watery diarrhoea in about 30% and 70% of cases respectively [112]. In some other studies, the proportion of *campylobacter* infections presenting as dysentery was much lower. In Guatemala, only 7 % of known *Campylobacter jejuni* infection presented with dysentery [113].

Yersinia enterocolitica grows at refrigerating temperature, hence, there is the risk of infection despite refrigeration of food materials. The exact mechanism of colonic invasion is unknown. However, the possession of enterotoxin genes and the production of heat-stable enterotoxins by the organism are indices of its virulence [114]. The production of cytokines and tumour necrosis factor and the impairment of nitric oxide secretion by macrophages may be ways by which the organism evades host defence mechanisms and causes the disease. The organism also presents as acute enteritis characterized by loose, bloody or watery stools which is usually self limiting in the older age group but may progress to bacteraemia in young infants.

Enteroinvasive *E. coli* (EIEC) shares a common virulence plasmid (pINV) with *Shigella* and thus, suspected to have a mechanism of cell invasion similar to that of *Shigella* [109]. During invasion, it attaches to the colonic enterocytes and enters the cells by endocytosis and thereafter multiply within the cytoplasm causing cell death and inflammatory response mediated by cytokines.

E. histolytica is transmitted when the infective cysts are ingested via foods and drinks contaminated with faecal matter, either by hands or by flies. These excyst in the colon releasing trophozoites which multiply repeatedly. Some of the trophozoites may form mononucleated cysts which later become tetra-nucleated infective cysts. These cysts do not excyst to form trophozoites again in the same host but when excreted in faeces, they may remain infective in sewage for many weeks. Trophozoites are not infective once passed out in faeces because they die rapidly but while they are still in the colon, they may become invasive, causing diseases like dysentery and amoebic liver abscess depending on the host immunity.

Amoebiasis follows within two weeks of infection with *E. histolytica* but it may be delayed for several months depending on the host's immunity [115]. The onset is usually gradual with tenesmus and frequent bowel motions usually, without remarkable constitutional symptoms. The stool is offensive and blood stained. It is acidic and usually contains both blood and mucus but scanty pus cells unlike in shigellosis where pus cells are profuse in the stools [115]. It may, on rare occasions, be complicated by toxic megacolon, intestinal perforation, peritonitis and amoeboma, which is a chronic form of amoebic colitis.

Tissue invasion only occurs in amoebiasis when the infecting strain is virulent as is the case in about 10% of cases of infection. When the organism is non-virulent, no mucosal invasion occurs and the infection remains asymptomatic even when amoebic cysts and non-haematophageous trophozoites are present in the faeces. The movement of the amoebic parasite for tissue invasion requires changes in parasite morphology and cytoskeletal dynamism which is provided by Myosin-IB, a motor protein constituent of the amoebic structure [116]. The trophozoites attach to the mucosa by galactose–specific lectins which are produced specifically to facilitate adhesion. They also release cysteine-rich proteases which degrade extracellular matrix components by histolysis and allow epithelial penetration. Peptides, phospholipases and haemolysins are then released to cause inflammation, tissue destruction, ulceration, exudation and increased stool liquidity.

Trichuris trichiura is transmitted faeco-orally and it inhabits the caecum and ascending colon. The mechanism of causing dysentery is however, unknown. Dysentery caused by *Trichuris* infestation also known as the *Trichuris* Dysentery Syndrome (TDS) only results from heavy *trichuris* infestation (defined as more than 10,000 eggs per gram of faeces) [117] since even occult gastrointestinal bleeding was absent in light trichuriasis. Infestation with this parasite is sometimes associated with a dysenteric illness known as the *Trichuris* Dysentery Syndrome (TDS) which is characterized by dysentery, stunting, anaemia and intellectual deficit. *Trichuris* Dysentery Syndrome typically presents with recurrent dysentery, stunting, anaemia, rectal prolapse, digital clubbing and intellectual deficit [118]. The growth failure in TDS may be a sequela of chronic inflammatory response in the intestinal mucosa. It is characterized by depressed plasma Insulin-like Growth Factor-1 and elevated tumour necrosis factor [119]. The former hormone is a growth enhancer while the latter suppresses appetite. Therefore, catch-up growth with increase in height and haemoglobin concentration had been reported to follow drug treatment of TDS but the mental deficit may persist [120].

Clinical Course and Complications

Passage of bloody loose stools characterized by urgency and tenesmus is the basic clinical feature of dysentery. This is shared by all the organisms known to cause dysentery such that it may be difficult to clinically distinguish the parasitic type from the bacillary type.

Shigellosis occurs about twelve hours after infection or much longer in some cases. It is characterized by tenesmus, high fever, emesis and anorexia [121]. At the onset, the stools are watery and profuse and later evolve into small, frequent, bloody and mucoid stools but this pattern changes often. Some patients may never reach the bloody stool stage while some may start with bloody stools from the onset. In shigellosis, the stool is odourless, watery and bloody, alkaline, and has numerous pus cells [81].

Shigellosis may be associated with severe dehydration or result in persistent diarrhoea. The complications of *shigella* dysentery may include, severe dehydration, hyponatraemia, syndrome of inappropriate antidiuretic hormone secretion, hypoglycaemia, protein losing enteropathy, and malnutrition [122]. Others include rectal prolapse, toxic megacolon, leukaemoid reaction, conjunctivitis, iritis, and arthritis [61]. Neurologic complications include seizures, headache, nuchal rigidity, hallucinations, lethargy, mutism and delirium. Explaining the seizures in shigellosis is difficult since *Shigella* meningitis is rare [61] and the fever in those who convulsed was not found to be unusually high, thereby making febrile seizure unlikely. Metabolic derangements like hyponatraemia and hypocalcaemia may be associated with seizures but they are not peculiar to shigellosis and seizures are not known with other forms of diarrhoeal diseases.

Shigellosis is characterized by raised serum levels of tumour necrosis factor (TNF) and nitric oxide (NO) but patients with neurologic complications have significantly higher levels of these substances [123]. This finding suggested that TNF and NO may play poorly defined roles in the pathogenesis of neurologic problems in shigellosis. Haemolytic uraemic syndrome complicating shigellosis may be due to shigatoxin mediated endothelial injury.

Dehydraton is unusual in dysentery and when it occurs it is regarded as a sign of severe illness. It is usually associated with *Shigella* dysentery especially due to *S. dysenteriae* type-1 strain.

Chapter VII

Persistent Diarrhoea

Most diarrhoeal episodes will resolve within 7 days but a few (about 20%) will be prolonged into and beyond the second week of the illness [124]. The World Health Organization recommended the term persistent diarrhoea for diarrhoea starting acutely as watery or bloody diarrhoea and lasting for at least fourteen days [2]. It is important to note that persistent diarrhoea does not encompass chronic diarrhoea which is also prolonged or recurrent diarrhoea most commonly due to non-infectious causes like endocrine, metabolic or nutritional disorders [2]. The clinical significance of persistent diarrhoea lies in the associated risk of malnutrition and mortality. Persistent diarrhoea forms between 30% and 50% of diarrhoeal deaths and the case-fatality-rate in persistent diarrhoea may be as high as 15% [1].

Persistent diarrhoea results from a combination of host, environmental and infectious factors which may include:

1. Young age – most cases of persistent diarrhoea occur in children age 24 months or less but mostly in infancy [125].
2. Recent measles infection – due to a combination of virus-induced mucosal damage and immune suppression which facilitate infection by other pathogens [126].
3. Inadequate or lack of breastfeeding due to poor intestinal epithelial protection [125,127].
4. High lactose concentration feeding has been shown to prolong the duration of illness.
5. Recent or prolonged antibiotic therapy alters intestinal flora predisposing to secondary infections [128].

6. Recent introduction of animal milk or formula as this may be associated with lactose intolerance or milk protein hypersensitivity which prolong diarrhoea [129].
7. Malnutrition – poor immune response delays the repair of gut epithelium causing prolongation of diarrhoea [125].
8. Vitamin A and Zinc deficiency are also associated with poor immune response to infection resulting in prolongation of diarrhoea [130].

On-going enteric infections cause villous flattening with mucosal damage. This encourages leakage of proteins into the submucosal tissue causing hypersensitivity, inflammation and hypersecretion. Thus, protein intolerance is central to the development of mucosal injury which results in persistent diarrhoea [131]. Common examples of proteins to which intolerance may develop include B-lactaglobulin in milk, soy-protein in soya beans and fish protein.

The same spectrum of enteropathogens is associated with both acute and persistent diarrhoea. It is important to note that more than one enteropathogen may be isolated in persistent diarrhoea and none may also be isolated. However, Rotavirus, *Aeromonas*, *Campylobacter*, enteroadherent *Escherichia coli*, *Salmonella*, *Shigella* and *Giardia* were reportedly associated with persistent diarrhoea in the developing world [132]. *Cryptosporidium parvum* was most commonly associated with persistent diarrhoea [133,134] while EAEC were the most important bacterial agents associated with persistent diarrhoea. The aggregative subgroups of EAEC were most common compared with the diffuse adhering EAEC (DA) and the localized adhering (LA) subgroups. In a cohort of Gambian children, ETEC was more significantly associated with persistent diarrhoea than EPEC [58]. However, a more recent multi-centre study reported enteropathogenic *E. coli* (EPEC) among 63% of children with persistent diarrhoea while viruses and parasites constituted less than 10% in that study [135]. The impact of persistent is heaviest on the nutritional status of children. Persistent diarrhoea occurs most frequently among undernourished children and commonly results in severe malnutrition. In addition, malnutrition is a leading cause of death in persistent diarrhoea.

Chapter IX

Chronic Diarrhoea

Chronic diarrhoea is uncommonly encountered in clinical practice especially in the developing world where most diarrhoeal episodes are infectious [6,131]. This disease is important because it is difficult to evaluate and manage especially in the under-resourced parts of the world where comprehensive laboratory investigation may be impossible. The rarity of chronic diarrhoea in the developing world may reflect the true epidemiology of the diseases associated with chronic diarrhoea or the lack of appropriate diagnostic facilities. Between 60 and 70% of chronic diarrhoea may be associated with malnutrition [10,131], while dehydration occurs in 39% of cases [10].

The aetiologies of chronic diarrhoea are numerous. Toddler's diarrhoea is non-specific diarrhoea which occurs in otherwise well toddlers especially within the age range of 6 to 24 months. The stools characteristically contain particles of undigested food. Although, the exact aetiology is unknown, toddler's diarrhoea is associated with dietary fat restriction and ingestion of poorly absorbed carbohydrates in fruit juices and carbonated drinks.

HIV enteropathy also presents with chronic diarrhoea which is a common presenting feature of childhood HIV/AIDS particularly in the tropics [136]. It is recognized as a major diagnostic and disease defining feature of paediatric HIV/AIDS in Africa [137]. HIV enteropathy is a syndrome of malabsorption with partial villous atrophy of non-infectious origin. It is postulated to result from direct invasion of the enterocytes by the HIV and destruction of the villi. Apart from this poorly-defined condition, chronic diarrhoea in HIV/AIDS may also be associated with enteropathogens like *Cryptosporidium parvum*, *Isospora belli* and *Enterocytozoon bieneusi* [138–140]. These enteropathogens cause prolonged diarrhoea from extensive intestinal mucosal damage. Notably, the same range of pathogens may be associated with diarrhoea among HIV-infected and HIV-uninfected children. These include ETEC, EAEC, *Shigella* and *Salmonella* [141,142]. Forty percent of chronic childhood diarrhoea in Tanzania had HIV seropositivity and remarkable association with parasitosis [143].

Post-enteritis syndrome results from transient mucosal damage which occurs during an acute enteric infection and is sustained thereafter. It is characterised by loss of digestive enzymes especially lactase resulting in lactose intolerance and osmotic diarrhoea. This condition was reported as the commonest aetiology of chronic childhood diarrhoea in Oman, [10] and Saudi Arabia, [131] but less common (10%) in Turkey [144].

Short bowel syndrome commonly follows surgical resection of a large proportion of the intestine. It may also occur secondary to congenital gastrointestinal malformation, Crohn's disease or necrotizing enterocolitis. This syndrome leads to alteration in normal intestinal motility resulting in intestinal fluid stasis, bacterial colonization, deconjugation of bile acids and inflammatory changes. The end result is malabsorption.

Malabsorption syndrome is a distinct clinical entity which is associated with chronic diarrhoea. Defects in the processes of digestion and absorption of nutrients result in chronic diarrhoea, abdominal distension and growth failure. Isolated single defects are rare hence multiple defects of absorption usually co-exist.

Malabsorption disorders are sub-divided into luminal, mucosal and intracellular defects. Luminal disorders which result in malabsorption include pancreatic insufficiency arising from chronic pancreatitis or cystic fibrosis. Two percent of the cases of chronic diarrhoea in Saudi Arabia had cystic fibrosis [131]. Schwachman's syndrome is another pancreatic exocrine disorder. It is associated with enzymatic defects in the absorption of carbohydrates, protein and fats. Giardiasis and cryptospiridosis are intestinal infestations which produce luminal disorders unrelated to pancreatic functions [144]. These parasitic infestations cause extensive villous destruction resulting in loss of brush border digestive enzymes and consequential malabsorption [145].

Mucosal defects which are associated with extensive reduction of the absorptive surface areas also result in malabsorption. Celiac disease is an example of this group of disorders and it formed between 13% and 30% of chronic childhood diarrhoea in Oman, Saudi Arabia and Turkey [10,131,144]. In Celiac's disease, exposure to gluten-containing foods results in extensive small intestine mucosal damage and villous atrophy. Decreased production of brush border enzymes like the disaccharidases and peptidases results in malabsorption. The exact mechanism in Celiac's disease is unknown but demonstration of anti-endomesial antibodies is diagnostic [146,147]. Malabsorption associated with colitis and chronic bloody diarrhoea also occurs in Cow's milk protein allergy. Acrodermatitis enteropathica which is, congenital zinc deficiency, was reported to cause 6% of chronic diarrhoea among Saudi Arabian children [131].

Intracellular defects following lack of intracellular digestive enzymes are relatively uncommon causes of malabsorption. These are followed by abnormal accumulation of the undigested nutrients and osmotic diarrhoea. The most common example of this group of defects is lactose intolerance resulting from lactase deficiency [131]. Others include sucrose-isomaltase deficiency, glucose-galactose malabsorption, congenital lipase deficiency, congenital trypsinogen deficiency, familial chloride diarrhoea, congenital enterokinase deficiency, intestinal lymphagiectasia and abetalipoprotein-aemia [131,148].

Conclusion

This book highlights the various types of diarrhoea peculiar to children with emphasis on the developing parts of the world where the burden of childhood diarrhoea is heaviest. Most of the cases of childhood diarrhoea are infectious and most of the causative organisms, otherwise known as enteropathogens, are acquired faeco-orally through contaminated foods, drinks and fingers. Therefore, the epidemiology of this condition is hinged on poor environmental sanitation, poor water supply and poor personal hygiene. Based on the data obtained from many parts of the world, it may be difficult to describe specific enteropathogens as commonest or rare. Bacterial and parasitic agents, hitherto regarded as uncommon causes of childhood diarrhoea, are now assuming premier positions in most parts of the developing world. Similarly, helminths and protozoans are also increasingly associated with childhood diarrhoea. More pathogens may in the future be identified as important pathogens in childhood diarrhoea. Infection with the Human Immunodeficiency Virus appears to have introduced an additional group of enteropathogens, albeit opportunistic agents, in childhood diarrhoea.

In addition, the evaluation of childhood diarrhoea needs to be improved in order to detect uncommon infectious cases as well as the non-infectious cases. Microbiological methods, including phenotyping of organisms, are being frequently reviewed for better efficiency. Further, serological methods are very helpful but have the major limitation of inability to clearly differentiate, frequently, between acute on-going and resolving infections. The implication of this is the need for health workers to have a good knowledge of the types and causes of diarrhoeal diseases peculiar to their locality of practice and be able to institute appropriate care. There is also a need for rapid diagnostic methods which could reliably detect enteropathogens with reliability and guide empirical treatment pending the availability of standard microbiological methods.

It is more important that improved environmental and personal hygiene would reduce the incidence as well as the burden of these diarrhoeal diseases.

References

[1] World Health Organization. World Health Statistics. 2009: 47 – 57.
[2] United Nations Children's Fund. Readings on diarrhoea. 1990.
[3] Bowie MD, Mann MD, Hill ID. A descriptive terminology of diarrhoeal diseases in infants and young children. *J. Trop. Pediatr.* 1992; 38: 55 - 56.
[4] World Health Organization. WHO Fact Sheet: Reducing mortality from major childhood killer diseases. *Fact Sheet Number* 180. 1997
[5] Mcremikwu MM, Asindi AA, Antia-Obong OE. The influence of breastfeeding on the occurrence of dysentery, persistent diarrhoea and malnutrition among Nigerian children with diarrhoea. *West Afr. J. Med.* 1997; 16: 20 – 23.
[6] Haque R, Mondal D, Kirkpatrick BD, Akther S, Farr BM, Sack RB, Petri WA Jr. Epidemiologic and clinical characteristics of acute diarrhoea with emphasis on Entamoeba histolytica infections in preschool children in an urban slum of Dhaka, Bangladesh. *Am. J. Trop. Med. Hyg.* 2003; 69: 398 – 405.
[7] Huilan S, Lu Guang Z, Mathan MM, Matthew MM, Olarte M, Espejo R *et al.* Etiology of acute diarrhoea among children in developing countries: a multicentre study in five countries. *Bull. World Health Org.* 1991; 69: 549 – 555.
[8] Haque R, Mondal D, Dugal P, Kabir M, Roy S, Farr M *et al.* Entamoeba histolytica infection in children and protection from subsequent amebiasis. *Infect. Immun.* 2006; 74: 904 – 909.
[9] Ogunlesi T, Okeniyi J, Oseni S, Oyelami O, Njokanma F, Dedeke O. Parasitic etiology of childhood diarrhoea. *Indian J. Pediatr.* 2006; 73: 1081 – 1084.

[10] Akinbami FO, Venugopalan P, Elnour IB, Nirmala V, Abiodun P, Azubuike JC. Pattern of chronic diarrhoea in children; a prospective analysis of causes, clinical features and outcome. *Niger. Postgrad. Med. J.* 2006; 13: 53 – 56.

[11] Imanzadeh F, Sayyeri AA, Yaghoobi M, Akbari MR, Shafagh H, Farsar AR. Celiac disease in children with diarrhoea is more frequent than previously suspected. *J. Pediatr. Gastroenterol. Nutr.* 2005; 40: 309 – 311.

[12] Shariff M, Deb M, Singh R. A study of diarrhoea among children in eastern Nepal with special reference to Rotavirus. *Indian J. M. Microbiol.* 2003; 21: 87 – 90.

[13] Synder JD, Merson MH. The magnitude of the global problem of acute diarrhoeal disease: a review of active surveillance data. *Bull. World Health Org.* 1992; 60: 605-3.

[14] Ekanem EE, Akitoye CO, Adedeji OT. Food hygiene behaviour and childhood diarrhoea in Lagos: a case-control study. *J. Diarrhoeal. Dis. Res.* 1991; 9: 219 - 226.

[15] Iroegbu CU, Ene-Obong HN, Uwaegbute AC, Amazigo UV. Bacteriological quality of weaning food and drinking water given to children of market women in Nigeria: implications for control of diarrhoea. *J. Health Popul. Nutr.* 2000; 18: 157 - 162.

[16] Gurgel RQ, Andrade JM, Machado-Neto P, Fabbro Al, Cuevas LE. Diarrhoea mortality in Aracaju, Brazil. *Ann. Trop. Paediatr.* 1997; 17: 361 - 365.

[17] Torres J, Gonzalez-Arroyo S, Perez R, Munoz O. Inappropriate treatment in children with bloody diarrhoea: clinical and microbiological studies. *Arch. Med. Res.* 1995; 26: 23 - 29.

[18] Wellington O, Chika O, Teslim O, Oladipo O, Adetayo F, Godswill I. Cryptosporidium and other intestinal protozoan in children with diarrhoea in Lagos, Nigeria. *The Internet Journal of Tropical Medicine.* 2009; Volume 5 Number 2. Available at http://www.ispub.com

[19] Djeneba O, Damintoti K, Denise I, Christelle NW, Virgillo P, Adrien B et al. Prevalence of rotavirus, adenovirus and enteric parasites among pediatric patients attending Saint Camille Medical Centre in Quagadougou. *Pak. J. Biol. Sci.* 2007; 10: 4266 – 4270.

[20] Carraturo A, Catalani V, Tega L. Microbiological and epidemiological aspects of rotavirus and enteric adenovirus infections in hospitalized children in Italy. *New Microbiol.* 2008; 31: 329 – 336.

References

[21] Abiodun PO. Incidence of rotavirus in acute diarrhoea in the University of Benin Teaching Hospital, Benin. *Nig. J. Paediatr.* 1989; 16: 31 – 34.

[22] Niyogi SK, Saha MR, De SP. Enteropathogens associated with acute diarrhoeal diseases. *Indian J. Public Health.* 1994; 38: 29 - 32.

[23] Mikhail IA, Hyams KC, Podgore JK *et al.* Microbiologic and clinical study of acute diarrhoea in children in Aswan, Egypt. *Scand. J. Infect. Dis.* 1989; 21: 59-65.

[24] Onyemelukwe NF. *Yersinia enterocolitica* as an aetiological agent of childhood diarrhoea in Enugu. *Cent. Afr. J. Med.* 1993; 39: 192 - 195.

[25] Odugbemi TO, Oyerinde JPO, Isaac-Sodeye JO, Roberts JIK. Parasitic and bacterial aetiology of childhood enteritis in Under-5. *West Afr. J. Med.* 1982; 1: 19-24.

[26] Ganong WF. Regulation of Gastrointestinal Function. In: Review of Medical Physiology. 22nd Edition. McGraw-Hill Company, New Delhi, 2005: 479 – 511.

[27] Mitchell RN, Kumar V, Abbas AK, Fausto N. Enterocolitis. In: Pocket Companion to Robbins and Cotran Pathologic Basis of Diseases. 7th Edition, Saunders Elsevier, Pennsylvania, 2006: 423 – 433.

[28] Sobel J, Gomes TA, Ramos RT, Hoekstra M *et al* Pathogen-specific risk factors and protective factors for acute diarrhoeal illness in children aged 12-59 months in Sao Paulo, Brazil. *Clin. Infect. Dis.* 2004; 38: 1545 - 1551.

[29] Knight SM, Toodayam W, Caique WC, Kyi W, Barnes A, Desmarchelier P. Risk factors for the transmission of diarrhoea in children: a case-control study in rural Malaysia. *Int. J. Epidemiol.* 1992; 21: 812 - 818.

[30] Oyedeji GA. The effect of socio-economic factors on the incidence and severity of gastroenteritis in Nigerian children. *Nig. Med. J.* 1987; 4: 229 – 232.

[31] Brown KH, Black RE, Robertson AD, Becker S. Effects of season and illness on the dietary intake of weanlings during longitudinal studies in rural Bangladesh. *Am. J. Clin. Nutr.* 1985; 41: 343 – 345.

[32] Roche N. Environmental Health. In: Lucas AO, Gilles HM (eds) Short Textbook of Public Health Medicine for the Tropics. Revised 4th Edition, Book Power, London, 2003: 337 – 352.

[33] Midzi SM, Tshimanga M, Siziya S, Marufu T, Mabiza ET. An outbreak of dysentery in a rural district of Zimbabwe: the role of personal hygiene at public gatherings. *Cent. Afr. J. Med.* 2000; 46: 150 – 153.

[34] Coward WA, Lunn PG. Biochemistry and physiology of kwashiorkor and marasmus. *Brit. Med. Bull.* 1981; 37: 19 – 24.
[35] Ogunlesi TA, Okeniyi JAO, Oyedeji OA, Njokanma OF, Aladekomo TA, Oyelami OA, Oyedeji GA. Home management of diarrhoea and dehydration among Nigerian children. *Nig. Med. Pract.* 2006; 50: 116 – 119
[36] Ogunlesi TA, Okeniyi JAO, Oyedeji OA, Oseni SBA, Oyelami OA, Njokanma OF. Childhood dysentery in Ilesa, Nigeria: The unusual role of Entamoeba histolytica. *The Internet Journal of Tropical Medicine.* 2005 Volume 2 Number 2. Available at http://www.ispub.com
[37] Thoren A, Stintzing G, Tufvesson B, Walder M, Habfe D. Aetiology and clinical features of severe infantile diarrhoea in Addis Ababa, Ethiopia. *J. Trop. Pediatr.* 1982; 28: 127 – 131.
[38] Kim KH, Suh IS, Kim JM, Kim CW, Cho YJ. Etiology of childhood diarrhoea in Korea. *J. Clin. Microbiol.* 1989; 27: 1192 – 1196.
[39] Ogunsanya TI, Rotimi VO, Adenuga A. A study of the aetiological agents of childhood diarrhoea in Lagos, Nigeria. *J. Med. Microbiol.* 1994; 40: 10 - 14.
[40] Orlandi PP, Silva T, Magalhaes GF, Alves F, Cunha RP, Durlacher R *et al*. Enteropathogens associated with diarrhoeal disease in infants of poor urban areas of Porto Velho, Rondonia: a preliminary study. *Mem. Inst. Oswaldo Cruz, Rio de Janeiro.* 2001; 96: 621 – 625.
[41] Manrique-Abril FG, Tigne Y, Diane B, Bello SE, Ospina JM. Diarrhoea-causing agents in children aged less than five years in Tunja, Colombia. *Rev. Salud Publica (Bogota).* 2006; 8: 88 – 97.
[42] Reither K, Ignatius R, Weitzel T, Seidu-Korkor A, Anyidoho L, Saad E *et al*. Acute childhood diarrhoea in northern Ghana: epidemiological, clinical and microbiological characteristics. *BMC Infectious Diseases* 2007, 7:104 doi:10.1186/1471-2334-7-104
[43] Simpore J, Ouermi D, Ilboudo D, Kabre A, Zeba B, Pietra V *et al*. Aetiology of acute gastro-enteritis inchildren at Saint Camille Medical Centre, Quagadougou, Burkina Faso. *Pak. J. Biol. Sci.* 2009; 12: 258 – 263.
[44] Mubashir M, Khan A, Baqai R, Iqbal J, Ghafoor A, Zuberi S, Burney MI. Causative agents of acute diarrhoea in the first 3 years of life: hospital-based study. *J. Gastroenterol. Hepatol.* 1990; 5: 264 – 270.
[45] Parashar UD, Gibson CJ, Bresee JS, Glass RI. Rotavirus and severe childhood diarrhoea. *Emerging Infect. Dis.* 2006; 12:304 – 306.

[46] Kim KH, Yang JM, Joo SI, Cho YG, Glass RI, Cho YJ. Importance of rotavirus and adenovirus types 40 and 41 in acute gastroenteritis in Korean children. *J. Clin. Microbiol.* 1990; 28: 2279 -2284.

[47] Medici MC, Martinelli M, Arcangelleti MC, Pinardi F, De Conto F, Dodi I et al. Epidemiological aspects of human rotavirus infection in children hospitalized with acute gastroenteritis in an area of northern Italy. *Acta Biomed.* 2004; 75: 100 -106.

[48] Black RE, Brown KH, Becker S, Abdul Alim ARM, Huq I. Longitudinal studies of infectious diseases and physical growth of children in rural Bangladesh. *Am. J. Epidemiol.* 1982; 115: 315 – 324.

[49] Audu R, Omilabu SA, Peenze I, Steele D. Viral diarrhoea in young children in two districts in Nigeria. *Cent. Afr. J. Med.* 2002; 48: 59 – 63.

[50] Fodha I, Chouikha A, Peenze I, De Beer M, Dewar J et al. Identification of viral agents causing diarrhoea among children in the Eastern Centre of Tunisia. *J. Med. Virol.* 2006; 78: 1198 – 1203.

[51] Abu-Elamreen FH, Abed AA, Shariff FA. Viral, bacterial and parasitic etiology of pediatric diarrhoea in Gaza, Palestine. *Med. Princ. Pract.* 2008; 17: 296 – 301.

[52] Orlandi PP, Magalhees GF, Matos NB, Silva T, Penatti M, Nogueira PA et al. Etiology of diarrhoeal infections in children of Porto Velho (Rondonia Western Amazon region, Brazil). *Braz. J. Med. Biol. Res.* 2006; 39: 507 – 517.

[53] Hien BT, Trang do T, Scheutz F, Cam PD, Malbak K, Dalsgaard A. Diarrhoegenic Escherichia coli and other causes of childhood diarrhoea: a case-control study in children living in a wastewater-use area in Hanoi, Vietnam. *J. Med. Microbiol.* 2007; 56: 1086 – 1096.

[54] Salem MB, Nadia HSB, Raja MNA. Bacterial aetiology and antimicrobial resistance of childhood diarrhoea in Yemen. *J. Trop. Pediatr.* 2001; 47: 301 – 302.

[55] Kain KC, Barteluk RL, Kelly MT, He X, de Hua G, Ge YA et al. Etiology of childhood diarrhoea in Beijing, China. *J. Clin. Microbiol.* 1991; 29: 90 – 95.

[56] Dosunmu-Ogunbi O, Coker AO, Agbonlahor DE, Solanke SO, Uzoma KC. Local pattern of acute enteric bacterial infections in man; -Lagos, Nigeria. *Dev. Biol. Stand.* 1983; 53: 277 - 283.

[57] Cohen N, Nataro J, Berstein D, Hawkins J, Roberts N, Staat M. Prevalence of diarrhoeagenic Escherichia coli in acute childhood enteritis: a prospective controlled study. *J. Pediatr.* 2005; 146: 54 – 61.

[58] Sullivan PB, Coles MAT, Aberra G, Ljungh A. Enteropathogenic and Enteroadherent- Escherichia coli in children with persistent diarrhoea and malnutrition. *Annals Trop. Paediatr.* 1994; 14: 105 – 110.

[59] Richie E, Punjabi NH, Corwin A, Lesmana M, Rogayah I, Lebron C et al. Enterotoxigenic Escherichia coli diarrhoea among young children in Jakarta, Indonesia. *Am. J. Trop. Med. Hyg.* 1997; 57: 85 – 90.

[60] Cavagnero F, Gana JC, Lagomarsino E, Vogel A, Gederlini A. Hemolytic-Uremic syndrome: the experience of a pediatric centre. *Rev. Med. Chil.* 2005; 133: 781 – 787.

[61] Barret-Connor E, Connor JD. Extraintestinal manifestations of shigellosis. *Am. J. Gastroenterol.* 1977; 4: 234 - 243.

[62] Patel PK, Mercy J, Shenoy J, Ashwini B. Factors associated with acute diarrhoea in children in Dhahira, Omani: a hospital-based study. *East Mediterr. Health J.* 2008; 14: 571 – 578.

[63] Sethi SK, Khuffah FA, al-Nakib W. Microbial aetiology of acute gastroenterology in hospitalized children in Kuwait. *Pediatr. Infect. Dis. J.* 1989; 8: 593 – 597.

[64] Ali M, Gheghesh KE, Aissa RB, Abuhelfaia A, Dufani M. Etiology of childhood diarrhoea in Zliten, Libya. *Saudi Med. J.* 2005; 26: 1759 – 1765.

[65] Wang SC, Chang LY, Hsueh PR, Lu CY, Lee PI, Shao PL et al. Campylobacter enteritis in children in northern Taiwan – a 7-year experience. *J. Microbiol. Immunol. Infect.* 2008; 41: 408 – 413.

[66] Puthucheary SD, Parasakthi N, Liew ST, Chee YW. Campylobacter enteritis in children: clinical and laboratory findings in 137 cases. *Singapore Med. J.* 1994; 35: 453 – 456.

[67] Bodhiatta L, Vithayasai N, Eimpokalarp B, Pitarangsi C, Serichantalergs O, Isenbarger DW. Bacterial enteric pathogens in children with acute dysentery in Thailand: increasing importance of quinolone-resistant Campylobacter. *Southeast Asian J. Trop. Med. Public Health* 2002; 33: 753 – 757.

[68] Soltan-Dallal MM, Moezardalan K. Frequency of Yersinia species infection in paediatric acute diarrhoea in Tehran. *East Mediterr. Health J.* 2004; 10: 152 – 158.

[69] Kanan TA, Abdulla ZA. Isolation of Yersinia spp from cases of diarrhoea in Iraqi infants and children. *East Mediterr. Health J.* 2009; 15: 276 – 284.

[70] Black RE, de Romana LG, Brown KH, Bravo N, Bazalar OG, Kanashiro HC. Incidence and etiology of infantile diarrhoea and major

routes of transmission in Huascar, Peru. *Am. J. Epidemiol.* 1989; 129: 785 – 799.

[71] Kehinde AO, Bakare RA, Oni AA, Okesola AO. Childhood gastroenteritis due to Aeromonas hydrophilia in Ibadan, Nigeria. *Afr. J. Med. Med. Sci.* 2001; 30: 345 – 346.

[72] Utsalo SJ, Eko FO, Antia-Obong OE, Nwaigwe CU. Aeromonads in acute diarrhoea and asymptomatic infection in Nigerian children. *Eur. J. Epidemiol.* 1995; 11: 171 – 175.

[73] Khan MA, Faruque ASG, Hossain G, Sattar S, Fuchs GJ, Salam MA. Plesiomonas shigelloides – associated diarrhoea in Bangladeshi children: A hospital-based surveillance study. *J. Trop. Pediatr.* 2004; 50: 354 – 356.

[74] Oyerinde JP, Ogunbi O, Alonge AA. Age and sex distribution of infections with *Entamoeba histolytica* and *Giardia intestinalis* in the Lagos population. *Int. J. Epidemiol.* 1977; 6: 231 - 234.

[75] Gonzalez-Ruiz A, Haque R, Aguirre A, Castandon G, Hall A, Guhl F *et al.* Value of microscopy in the diagnosis of dysentery associated with invasive Entamoeba histolytica. *J. Clin. Pathol.* 1994; 47: 236 – 239.

[76] Adamu H, Endeshaw T, Teka T, Kifle A, Pettros B. The prevalence of intestinal parasites in paediatric diarrhoeal and non-diarrhoeal patients in Addis Ababa hospitals with special emphasis on opportunistic parasitic infections and with insight into the demographic and socio-economic factors. *Ethiopian J. Health Dev.* 2005; 20: 39 – 46.

[77] Pereira MC, Atwill ER, Barbosa AP. Prevalence and associated risk factors for Giardia lamblia infection among children hospitalized for diarrhoea in Goiania, Goias State, Brazil. *Rev. Inst. Med. Trop. S. Paulo.* 2007; 49: 139 – 145.

[78] Chintu C, Luo C, Baboo S, Khumalo-Ngwenya B, Mathewson J, DuPontn HL *et al.* Intestinal parasites in HIV-positive Zambian children with diarrhoea. *J. Trop. Pediatr.* 1995; 41: 149 – 152.

[79] Eden OB. Neuroblastoma. In: Hendrickse RG, Barr DGD, Matthews TS (eds.) Paediatrics in the Tropics. 1st Edition. Blackwell Scientific Publications, Oxford. 1991: 563 - 564.

[80] Kuskonmaz B, Yurdakok K, Yalcin SS, Ozmert E. Comparison of acute bloody and watery diarrhoea: a case-control study. *Turk J. Pediatr.* 2009; 51: 133 – 140.

[81] Mathan VI, Mathan MM. Intestinal manifestations of invasive diarrhoea and their diagnosis. *Rev. Infect. Dis.* 1991;13 (Suppl 4) : S311 – S313.

[82] Knight R. Intestinal parasites and host susceptibility in children. In: Hendrickse RG (ed.) Paeditrics in the Tropics. Current Review.1st Edition.ELBS/Oxford University Press, Oxford. 1985: 326 - 327.
[83] Banerjee B, Hazra S, Bandyopadhyay D. Diarrhoea management among under-fives. *Indian Pediatr.* 2004; 41: 255 - 260.
[84] Malakooti MA, Alaii J, Shanks GD, Phillips-Howard PA. Epidemic dysentery in Western Kenya. *Trans. R. Soc. Trop. Med. Hyg.* 1997; 91: 541 - 543.
[85] Engels D, Madaras T, Nyandwi S, Murray J. Epidemic dysentery caused by *Shigella dysenteriae* type-1: a sentinel site surveillance of antimicrobial resistance patterns in Burundi. *Bull. World Health Org.* 1995; 73: 787 - 791.
[86] World Health Organisation. The treatment of diarrhoea. A manual for Physicians and Other Senior Health Workers. WHO/CDD/95.3: 1995
[87] Rawashdeh OM, Ababneh AM, Shurman AA. Shigellosis in Jordanian children:a clinico-epidemiological prospective study and susceptibility to antibiotics. *J. Trop. Pediatr.* 1994; 40: 355 - 359.
[88] Taylor DN, Echeverria P, Pitarangsi P, Seriwatana J, Bodhidatta L, Blaser MJ. Influence of strains characteristics and immunity on the epidemiology of campylobacter infections in Thailand. *J. Clin. Microbiol.* 1988; 26: 863 – 868.
[89] Duguid JP, Marmion BP, Swain RHA. *Salmonella* In: Duguid JP, Marmion BP, Swain RHA (eds.) Mackie and McCartey Medical Microbiology Volume 1. 13th Edition, ELBS/Churchill Livingstone. Edinburgh 1985; 320 - 322.
[90] Albert MJ, Faruque SM, Sack RB, Mahalanabis D. Case-control study of enteropathogens associated with childhood diarrhoea in Dhaka, Bangladesh. *J. Clin. Microbiol.* 1999; 37: 3458 - 3464.
[91] Niyogi SK, Saha MR, De SP. Enteropathogens associated with acute diarrhoeal diseases. *Indian J. Public Health.* 1994; 38: 29-32.
[92] Nathoo KJ, Mason PR, Trijssenaar FL, Lyons NF, Tswana SA. Microbial pathogens associated with diarrhoea in children admitted to Harare Hospital for rehydration therapy. *Cent. Afr. J. Med.* 1986; 32: 118 - 123.
[93] Carniel E, Butler T, Hossain S, Alam NH, Mazigh D. Infrequent detection of *Yersinia enterocolitica* in childhood diarrhoea in Bangladesh. *Am. J. Trop. Med. Hyg.* 1986; 35: 370 - 371.
[94] Youssef M, Shurman A, Bougnoux M, Rawashdeh M, Bretagne S, Strockbine N. Bacterial, viral and parasitic enteric pathogens associated with acute diarrhoea in hospitalized children from northern

Jordan. *FEMS (Federation of European Microbiological Societies) Immunol. Med. Microbiol* 2000; 28: 257- 263.

[95] Dutta S, Chatterjee A, Dutta P, Rajendram K, Roy S, Pramanik KC, Bhattacharya SK. Sensitivity and performance characteristics of a direct PCR with stool samples in comparison to conventional techniques for diagnosis of *Shigella* and enteroinvasive *Escherichia coli* infection in children with acute diarrhoea in Calcutta, India. *J. Med. Microbiol* 2001; 50: 667- 674.

[96] Ihekwaba FN. Abdominal *Tuberculosis*: a study of 881 cases. *J. R. Coll. Surg. Edinburgh* 1993; 38: 293 - 295.

[97] Fisher MC. Pseudomembranous Colitis. In: Behrman RE, Kliegman RM, Jenson HB (eds.) Nelson's Textbook of Pediatrics, 16th Edition, WB Saunders Company, Pennsylvania.2000: 881.

[98] World Health Organization. Amoebiasis. WHO Weekly Epidemiologic Record 1997; 72: 97 – 100.

[99] Weissman SB, Salata RA. Amoebiasis. In: Behrman RE, Kliegman RM, Jenson HB (eds.) Nelson's Textbook of Pediatrics, 16th Edition, WB Saunders Company, Pennsylvania. 2000: 1035 - 1036.

[100] Shetty N, Narasinha M, Elliot E, Raj IS, Macaden R. Age-specific seroprevalence of amoebiasis and giardiasis in southern Indian infants and children. *J. Trop. Pediatr.* 1992; 38: 57 - 62.

[101] Ighogboja IS, Ikeh EI. Parasitic agents in childhood diarrhoea and malnutrition. *West Afr. J. Med.* 1997; 16: 36 - 39.

[102] Yakubu AM, Bello CSS. Bacterial and parasitic agents in diarrhoeal stools in Zaria. *Postgraduate Doctor Africa.* 1988; 10: 249 - 250.

[103] Wyllie R. Intussusception. In: Behrman RE, Kliegman RM, Jenson HB (eds.) Nelson's Textbook of Pediatrics, 16th Edition, WB Saunders Company, Pennsylvania.2000: 1142 - 1143.

[104] Buller HA. Problems in diagnosis in Inflammatory Bowel Disease in children. *Neth. J. Med.* 1997; 50: S8 – S11.

[105] Gryboski JD. Ulcerative colitis in children 10 years old or younger. *J. Pediatr. Gastroenterol. Nutr.* 1993; 17: 24 – 31.

[106] Ulshen M. Inflammatory Bowel Diseases. In: Behrman RE, Kliegman RM, Jenson HB (eds.) Nelson's Textbook of Pediatrics, 16th Edition, WB Saunders Company, Pennsylvania.2000: 1150 - 1157.

[107] Gomez HF, Cleary TG. *Shigella*. In: Behrman RE, Kliegman RM, Jenson HB (eds.) Nelson's Textbook of Pediatrics, 16th Edition, WB Saunders Company, Pennsylvania. 2000; 848 - 849.

[108] Cam PD, Adii R, Lindberg AA, Pal T. Antibodies against invasion plasmid coded antigens of *Shigella* in human colostrums and milk. *Acta Microbiologica Hungrica*. 1992; 39: 263 - 270.
[109] Prats G, Llovet T. Enteroinvasive *Escherichia coli*: Pathogenesis and epidemiology. (Spanish). *Microbiologia*. 1995; 11: 91- 96.
[110] Nhieu GT, Sansonetti PJ. Mechanism of *Shigella* entry into epithelial cells. *Current Opinion in Microbiology*.1999; 2: 51- 55.
[111] Francois M, Le Cabec V, Dupont MA, Sansonetti PJ, Maridonneau-Parini I. Induction of necrosis in human neutrophils by *Shigella flexneri* requires type III secretion, IpaC invasions and actin polymerization. *Infect. Immun.* 2000; 68: 1289 - 1296.
[112] Skirrow MB. *Campylobacter* enteritis. Postgraduate-Doctor Africa 1985; 7:165 - 168.
[113] Ramiro Cruz J, Cano F, Bartlett AV, Mendez H. Infection, diarrhoea and dysentery caused by *Shigella* species and *Campylobacter jejuni* among Guatemalan children. *Pediatr. Inf. Dis. J.* 1994; 13: 216 - 223.
[114] Singh I, Virdi JS. Production of *Yersinia* stable toxin (YST) and distribution of yst genes in biotype 1A strains of *Yersinia enterocolitica*. *J. Med. Microbiol*. 2004; 53: 1065 - 1068.
[115] Weissman SB, Salata RA. Amoebiasis. In: Behrman RE, Kliegman RM, Jenson HB (eds.) Nelson's Textbook of Pediatrics, 16th Edition, WB Saunders Company, Pennsylvania. 2000: 1035 - 1036.
[116] Reed S, Bouvier J, Polleck AS *et al*. Cloning of a virulence factor of *E. histolytica*. Pathogenic strains possess a unique cysteine proteinase gene. *J. Clin. Invest*. 1993; 91: 1532 - 1540.
[117] Raj SM. Fecal occult blood testing on *Trichuris*-infected primary school children in northeastern Peninsular Malaysia. *Am. J. Trop. Med. Hyg*. 1999; 60: 165 - 166.
[118] Kazura JW. *Trichuris*. In: Behrman RE, Kliegman RM, Jenson HB (eds.) Nelson's Textbook of Pediatrics, 16th Edition, WB Saunders Company, Pennsylvania.2000: 1073.
[119] Duff EM, Andeson NM, Cooper ES. Plasma insulin-like growth factor-1, type-1 procollagen and serum tumour necrosis factor-alpha in children recovering from *Trichuris* Dysentery Syndrome. *Pediatr*. 1999; 103: e69.
[120] Callender JE, Grantham-McGregor SM, Walker Sp, Cooper ES. Treatment effects in *Trichuris* Dysentery Syndrome. *Acta Paediatr*. 1994; 83: 1182 - 1187.
[121] Sirivichayakul C, Thisyakorn U. Severe shigellosis in childhood. *South-eastern Asian J Trop Med Public Health*. 1998; 29: 555 - 559.

[122] Gomez HF, Cleary TG. *Shigella*. In: Behrman RE, Kliegman RM, Jenson HB (eds.) Nelson's Textbook of Pediatrics, 16th Edition, WB Saunders Company, Pennsylvania. 2000; 848 - 849.

[123] Mor M, Yuhas Y, Kaminsky E, Dinari G, Ashkenazi S. Induction of tumour necrosis factor and nitric oxide by *Shigella* strains isolated from patients with or without neurologic manifestations. *Israel J. Med. Sci.* 1996; 32: 1271 - 1275.

[124] Bhan MK, Arora NK, Khoshoo V, Ghai OP. Chronic diarrhoea in infants and children. *Indian J. Pediatr.* 1985; 53: 483 – 495.

[125] Ahmed M, Billo AG, Murtaza G. Risk factors for persistent diarrhoea in children below five years of age. *J. Pak. Med. Assoc.* 1995; 45: 290 – 292.

[126] Feachem RG, Koblinsky MA. Interventions for the control of diarrhoeal diseases among children: mealse immunization. *Bull. World Health Org.* 1983; 61: 641 – 652.

[127] Brown KH, Black RE, Lopez de Romana G, Kanashiro HC. Infant feeding practices and their relationship with diarrhoeal and other diseases in Huascar (Lima) Peru. *Pediatr.* 1989; 83: 31 – 40.

[128] Harris S, Black RE. How useful are pharmaceuticals in managing diarrhoeal diseases in the developing countries. *Health Policy and Planning.* 1991; 6: 141 – 147.

[129] Brown HA, Lake A. Appropriate use of human and non-human milks for the dietary management of children with diarrhoea. *J. Diarrhoea Dis. Res.* 1991; 9: 168 – 185.

[130] Beisel WR. Single nutrients and immunity. *Am. J. Clin. Nutr.* 1982; 35: 417 – 468.

[131] Abdullah M. Aetiology of chronic diarrhoea in children: experience at King Khalid University Hospital, Riyadh, Suadi Arabia. *Ann. Trop. Paediatr.* 1994; 14: 111 – 117.

[132] Henry FJ, Udoy AS, Wanke CA, Aziz K. Epidemiology of persistent diarrheoa and etiologic agents in Mirzapur, Bangladesh. *Acta Paediatr.* 1991; 81: 27 – 31.

[133] Shaheen S, Shoaib T, Amtul H. Frequency of Cryptosporidium in childhood diarrhoea – Importance of Modified Acid Fast Technique. Available at http://www.ayubmed.edu.pk/ JAMC/ PAST/15-3/Shaheenshuaib.htm

[134] Araya M, Espinoza J, Pacheco I, Altieri AM, Brunser O. Cryptospiridosis: Studies in children in communities of low socioeconomic level. *Rev. Chil Pediatr.* 1990; 61: 262 – 267.

[135] Abba K, Sinfield R, Hart CA, Garner P. Pathogens associated with persistent diarrhoea in children inlow and middle income countries: systematic review. *BMC Infectious Diseases*. 2009. 9:88 doi: 10.1186/1471-2334-9-88.

[136] Emodi IJ, Okafor GO. Child manifestations of HIV infants in children at Enugu, Nigeria. *J. Trop. Pediatr.* 1998; 44: 73 – 76.

[137] African Network for the Care of Children affected by HIV/AIDS. Handbook on Paediatric AIDS in Africa for Medical students, Doctors and Primary Care Workers. 2004.

[138] Amadi B, Kelly P, Mwiya M, Mulwazi E, Sianongo S, Changwe F et al. Intestinal and systemic infection with HIV and mortality in Zambian children with persistent diarrhoea and malnutrition. *J. Pediatr. Gastroenterol. Nutr.* 2001; 32: 550 – 554.

[139] Bretagne S, Foulet F, Alkassoum W, Fleury-Feith J, Develoux M. Prevalence of Enterocytozoon bieneusi spores in the stool of AIDS patients and African children not infected by HIV. *Bull. Soc. Pathol. Exot.* 1993; 86: 351 – 357.

[140] Barboni G, Candi M, Ines Villace M, Leonardelli A, Balbaryski J, Gaddi E. Intestinal cryptosporidiosis in HIV-infected children. *Medicina (B Aires)*. 2008; 68: 213 – 218.

[141] Muslime V, Kalyesubula I, Kaddu-Mulindwa D, Byarugaba J. Enteric bacterial pathogens in HIV-infected children with acute diarrhoea in Mulago Referral and Teaching Hospital, Kampala, Uganda. *Journal of the International Association of Physicians in AIDS Care.* 2009; 8: 185 – 190.

[142] Kakai R, Bwayo JJ, Plummer FA. Enteric pathogens and severity of diarrhoea in HIV infected children. *Int. Conf. AIDS.* 1993; 9: 6 – 11.

[143] Cegielski P, Msengi AE, Dukes CS, Mbise R, Redding-Lallinger R, Minjas JN et al. Intestinal parasites and HIV infection in Tanzanian children with chronic diarrhoea. *AIDS.* 1993; 7: 213 – 221.

[144] Altuntas B, Gul H, Yarali N, Ertan N. Etiology of chronic diarrhoea. *Indian J. Pediatr.* 1999; 66: 657 – 661.

[145] Buret AG. Pathology of enteric infections with Giardia duodenalis. *Parasite.* 2008; 15: 261 – 265.

[146] Bhatnager S, Gupta SD, Mathur M, Phillips AD, Kumar R, Knutton S et al. Celiac disease with mild to moderate histologic changes is a common cause of chronic diarrhoea in indian children. *J. Pediatr. Gastroenterol. Nutr.* 2005; 41: 204 – 209.

[147] Canales RP, Araya MQ, Alliende GF, Hunter MB, Alarcon OT, Chavez SE. Diagnosis and clinical presentation of Celiac disease: a multicentre study. *Rev. Med. Chil.* 2008; 136: 296 – 303.

[148] Belmont JW, Reid B, Taylor W, Baker SS, Moore WH, Morriss MC *et al*. Congenital sucrase-isomaltase deficiency presenting with failure to thrive, hypercalcaemia and nephrocalcinosis. *BMC Pediatr.* 2002; 2:4.

Reviewed by: Prof. Fidelis O. Njokanma of the Department of Paediatrics and Child Health, Lagos State University College of Medicine, Ikeja, Lagos, Nigeria.

Index

A

acid, 7
acidity, 10
active transport, 7
adenovirus, 13, 36, 39
adhesion, 23, 24
adolescents, 21
adrenogenital syndrome, 18
aetiology, 19, 22, 29, 30, 37, 39, 40
Africa, 20, 29, 43, 44, 46
age, 5, 20, 24, 27, 29, 45
AIDS, viii, 29, 46
Aldrich syndrome, 18
allergy, 31
alters, 27
amebiasis, 35
anorexia, 25
antibiotic, 11, 27
antidiuretic hormone, 26
antigen, 17
antimicrobial therapy, 21
appetite, 25
arthritis, 26
ascending colon, 25
asymptomatic, 17, 21, 24, 41
atrophy, 10, 29, 30
availability, 11, 34

B

bacteria, vii, 11
bacterial infection, 39
Bangladesh, 12, 13, 15, 17, 19, 20, 35, 37, 39, 42, 45
Beijing, 39
bile, 30
bile acids, 30
bleeding, 25
blood, vii, 3, 7, 17, 19, 24, 44
blood vessels, 7
bowel, 22, 24, 30
Brazil, 12, 15, 36, 37, 39, 41
breast milk, 9, 10, 22
breastfeeding, 9, 10, 22, 27, 35
Burkina Faso, 12, 38

C

caecum, 25
campylobacter, 23, 42
carbohydrates, 29, 30
carcinoid syndrome, viii, 18
carrier, 21
causation, 11
cell death, 23, 24
cell invasion, 24
cell surface, 23

central nervous system, 14
chicken, 23
China, 12, 39
classes, 11
cleaning, 10
clinical disorders, 15
clinical presentation, 47
clubbing, 25
cohort, 9, 15, 16, 20, 21, 28
colic, 1
colitis, 22, 24, 31, 43
Colombia, 12, 38
colon, 21, 24, 25
colonization, 10, 30
colostrum, 22
coma, 15
community, vii
complications, 25, 26
components, 25
concentration, 7, 8, 25, 27
conjunctivitis, 26
contamination, 9
control, 36, 37, 39, 41, 42, 45
CSS, 43
culture, 20
cyst, 17
cystic fibrosis, 30
cytokines, 22, 23, 24
cytoplasm, 24

D

deaths, 1, 5, 13, 17, 19, 23, 24, 27, 28
defects, 18, 30, 31
defence, 24
deficiency, viii, 18, 28, 31, 47
deficit, 5, 25
dehydration, 13, 14, 17, 19, 25, 29, 38
delirium, 26
depolymerization, 23
destruction, 25, 29, 30
detection, 42
developing countries, 20, 35, 45
dietary fat, 29
dietary intake, 37
digestion, 30
digestive enzymes, 8, 30, 31
disorder, 30
distribution, 41, 44
dogs, 23
drinking water, 36
drug treatment, 25
drugs, 8
duodenum, 17
duration, 19, 27
dynamism, 24

E

East Asia, 1
economic status, 9
Egypt, 5, 37
electrolyte, 5
endocrine, viii, 27
endocrine disorders, viii
enteritis, viii, 24, 30, 37, 38, 39, 40, 44
enterokinase, 31
enzymes, 8, 30, 31
epidemic, 19, 20
epidemiology, 29, 33, 42, 44
epithelial cells, 7, 8, 23, 44
epithelium, viii, 8, 23, 28
erosion, 23
etiology, viii, 35, 39, 40
exotoxins, 14, 18
exposure, 30
extracellular matrix, 25

F

failure, 25, 30, 47
failure to thrive, 47
family, 9
fasting, 8
fat, 29
febrile seizure, 26
fever, 13, 25, 26

fibrosis, 30
fish, 28
flatulence, 17
flora, 10, 21, 27
fluid, 5, 7, 8, 18, 22, 30
food, 9, 18, 23, 29, 36

G

gastroenteritis, 37, 39, 41
gastrointestinal bleeding, 25
gastrointestinal tract, 10, 13, 14
genes, 23, 44
glucose, 7, 31
grades, 8
growth, 21, 25, 30, 39, 44
Guatemala, 23
gut, viii, 7, 10, 14, 16, 17, 18, 21, 22, 23, 28

H

hallucinations, 26
hands, 24
headache, 26
health, 33
heat, 14, 16, 23
height, 25
HIV, viii, 17, 29, 41, 46
hormone, 25, 26
hospitalization, vii, 13
hospitals, 41
host, 24, 27, 42
HSB, 39
human milk, 45
human neutrophils, 44
Hunter, 47
hydrogen, 7
hygiene, 9, 33, 34, 36, 37
hyperparathyroidism, 18
hypersensitivity, 28

I

idiopathic, 22
ileum, 20
immune response, 10, 28
immunity, 24, 42, 45
immunization, 45
immunocompromised, 17
immunodeficiency, 18
immunoglobulins, 9
immunosuppression, viii
incidence, 5, 9, 34, 37
income, 46
India, 5, 12, 19, 20, 21, 43
indices, 23
Indonesia, 40
infancy, 5, 13, 22, 27
infants, 1, 5, 9, 13, 20, 22, 24, 35, 38, 40, 43, 45, 46
infection, 10, 13, 15, 17, 20, 23, 24, 25, 27, 28, 30, 35, 39, 40, 41, 43, 46
infectious disease, 39
infestations, 6, 22, 30
inflammation, 17, 18, 22, 23, 25, 28
inflammatory bowel disease, 22
inflammatory disease, 19
inflammatory mediators, 22
ingestion, 18, 29
injury, 26, 28
insects, 9
insulin, 44
intestinal flora, 27
intestinal perforation, 24
intestine, 7, 17, 30
intussusception, 22
ions, 7
iritis, 26
iron, 18
isolation, 5, 11, 12, 13, 14, 15, 16, 17
Israel, 45
Italy, 36, 39

J

jejunum, 17
Jordan, 20, 21, 43

K

Kenya, 42
Korea, 12, 38
Kuwait, 40

L

lactase, 30, 31
lactose, viii, 10, 27, 28, 30, 31
lactose intolerance, viii, 10, 28, 30, 31
large intestine, 7
leakage, 28
lethargy, 26
likelihood, 9, 12
limitation, 33
liquidity, 23, 25
liver abscess, 24
lumen, 7, 8, 14, 17, 19

M

macrophages, 9, 24
malabsorption, viii, 29, 30, 31
malaria, 12
Malaysia, 20, 37, 44
malnutrition, 10, 14, 21, 26, 27, 28, 29, 35, 40, 43, 46
management, 38, 42, 45
market, 36
mast cells, 23
matrix, 25
measles, 12, 27
Mediterranean, 1
membranes, 23
meningitis, 26
Mexico, 12
microscopy, 41
milk, viii, 9, 10, 22, 28, 31, 44
morbidity, 1, 19
morphology, 24
mortality, 1, 19, 27, 35, 36, 46
movement, 8, 24
mucoid, 25
mucosa, 24, 25
mucus, 19, 24
Myanmar, 12

N

necrosis, 19, 23, 25, 26, 44, 45
Nepal, 36
nephrocalcinosis, 47
nervous system, 14
neuroblastoma, 18
neutrophils, 44
Nigeria, 5, 12, 13, 16, 20, 21, 36, 38, 39, 41, 46, 47
nitric oxide, 23, 26, 45
nuchal rigidity, 26
nutrients, 30, 31, 45

O

occult blood, 17, 44
order, 33
organism, 14, 15, 16, 17, 21, 23, 24
osmolality, 8
oxygen, 22

P

Pacific, 1
pain, 17
Pakistan, 12
pancreatic insufficiency, viii, 30
pancreatitis, 30
parasite, 17, 24, 25
parasitic infection, 41
particles, 29

pathogenesis, 26
pathogens, vii, 9, 10, 11, 12, 13, 14, 27, 30, 33, 40, 42, 46
PCR, 43
pellagra, 18
peptides, 18
perforation, 24
peristalsis, 8
peritonitis, 24
personal hygiene, 9, 33, 34, 37
Peru, 41, 45
phagocytosis, 23
pharmaceuticals, 45
pheochromocytoma, 18
physiology, 7, 38
plasma, 25
plasmid, 22, 23, 24, 44
pneumonia, 12
polymerase chain reaction, 12
polymerization, 44
polyps, 22
poor, 5, 9, 18, 27, 28, 33, 38
population, 17, 21, 41
preschool, 35
preschool children, 35
primary school, 44
production, 7, 10, 23, 30
prolapse, 25, 26
prostaglandins, 22
protective factors, 37
proteinase, 44
proteins, 28
pus, 8, 24, 25

R

range, 29, 30
rectal prolapse, 25, 26
region, 39
rehydration, 42
relapses, 22
relationship, 9, 45
reliability, 34
repair, 28
resection, 30
resistance, 39, 42
respiratory, 13
risk, 5, 9, 10, 14, 23, 27, 37, 41
risk factors, 37, 41
rotavirus, 5, 13, 36, 37, 39

S

Saudi Arabia, 30
school, 44
scleroderma, viii
secretion, 7, 8, 14, 18, 22, 23, 26, 44
seizure, 26
serology, vii, 21
serum, 26, 44
severity, 37, 46
sewage, 9, 21, 23, 24
sex, 41
shigella, 25
shock, 17
Singapore, 40
small intestine, 17, 30
sodium, 7, 8
Southeast Asia, 40
species, 8, 14, 15, 16, 17, 20, 21, 22, 40, 44
spectrum, 28
stasis, 30
strain, 24, 26
students, 46
subgroups, 14, 16, 28
substrates, 8
sucrose, 31
supply, 9, 33
suppression, 27
surface area, 7, 8, 30
surgical resection, 30
surveillance, 36, 41, 42
susceptibility, 42
symptoms, 24
syndrome, viii, 14, 15, 18, 25, 26, 29, 30, 40

T

Taiwan, 40
Tanzania, 30
temperature, 23
Thailand, 40, 42
therapy, 21, 27, 42
thyrotoxicosis, 18
tissue, 23, 24, 28
TNF, 26
toddlers, 29
toxic megacolon, 24, 26
toxin, 14, 18, 22, 44
traits, 22
transmission, 13, 37, 41
transport, 7
Turkey, 30

U

ulcerative colitis, 22
United Nations, 35
urban areas, 38

V

vacuole, 23
vasoactive intestinal peptide, 18
vessels, 7
Vietnam, 13, 39
viral infection, 22
viruses, vii, 11, 13, 28
vomiting, 13, 19

W

waste disposal, 9
wastewater, 39
water supplies, 9
women, 36
workers, 33
World Health Organisation, 42

Y

Yemen, 39

Z

Zimbabwe, 37
zinc, viii, 31